Fracture Classifications
in Clinical Practice

T0235906

Seyed Behrooz Mostofi

Fracture Classifications in Clinical Practice

Second Edition

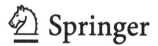

Seyed Behrooz Mostofi FRCS (Tr&Orth)
Consultant Orthopaedic Surgeon
Kent and Canterbury Hospital
Canterbury
Kent, UK

ISBN 978-1-4471-4419-9   ISBN 978-1-4471-4420-5   (eBook)
DOI 10.1007/978-1-4471-4420-5
Springer London Heidelberg New York Dordrecht

Library of Congress Control Number: 2012954866

Printed on acid-free paper

Springer is part of Springer Science+Business Media (www.springer.com)

*This book is dedicated in loving memory of my
grandparents:*

*Mr. Seyed Abbas Mostofi, philosopher, poet, writer
and diplomat, who devoted his life to the education,
happiness and well being of others
and
Mrs. Khadijeh Mostofi, a lady of influential status,
far in advance of her time, who insisted that strong
moral values and a high standard of spiritual belief
be maintained in her family.*

God bless them.

Foreword

This is one of those necessary books to which one rushes to confirm that one's memory of fracture classification is correct. It is succinctly written and well referenced, providing a quick and easy aide memoir of fracture patterns. Drawn from many sources, a number of classifications are usefully provided for each fracture area.

Whether as a useful introduction to trauma, or as an essential prior to examination, with this book Behrooz Mostofi has produced a little gem.

Barry Hinves
Chair, Specialist Training Committee
South East Thames Rotation
University of London
United Kingdom

Preface to the Second Edition

It has been over 7 years since the first edition of this book appeared. During that time it was well received all over the world and was translated into Portuguese and Chinese. I was humbled by the flood of appreciation notes from doctors, students, residents, and all those preparing for professional examinations. This has been a most gratifying feeling.

Under these circumstances, it is to be expected that in a second edition of a book like *Fracture Classifications in Clinical Practice* there would need to be some revision if it is to continue to address the needs of an international audience. For the new edition, I have made many changes and have added a number of additional classifications and diagrams.

It has been a pleasure working again with the Springer publication team, in particular and my editor, Steffan Clements.

I hope you will enjoy reading this new edition and benefit from the additional material.

Seyed Behrooz Mostofi
Canterbury
May 2012

Preface to the First Edition

Staff in accident and emergency department and doctors in fracture clinic alike may at times find themselves that they are inadequately equipped to identify the exact type of a given fracture unless they have access to a text book.

Classification is an essential aid, which guide the clinical judgment. It has been developed to facilitate organization of seemingly distinct but related fracture into different clinically useful groups. Ideally it should provide a reliable language of communication, guideline for a treatment, and to allow a reasonable progress to be drawn for a specific type of fracture. However, the "ideal" classification system does not exist to fulfill the entire requirement needed from such a scheme. As a result there are numerous classification systems for each fractures published in the literature; some more used in one continent than others.

This book makes no attempt to produce a comprehensive list of all classifications. I have endeavored to include those systems that are practical and proven to be helpful in everyday clinical practice by a majority of surgeons. The aim of this book is to give enough essentials to take the major task of identification and analysis of fracture, which is the first step in treatment of fracture patients.

Even as more system of classification will evolve in time, the likelihood that classifications appeared in this book would continue to provide guidance in fracture care far into the future remains high. I accept responsibility for any short-comings in this book and corrections will be gladly made in the next edition

Seyed Behrooz Mostofi
London
August 2005

Acknowledgments

I am grateful to Dr. Andrée Bates whose unfailing support is a source of inspiration.

I acknowledge the help and advice of my old friend, and talented orthopedic surgeon, Mr. H. Khairandish (Payman), from whom I have benefited enormously.

I am indebted to Mr. Ravi Singh for his encouragement and suggestions at the times most needed.

I would like to give special thanks to Grant Weston, Hannah Wilson, Barbara Chernow, and other staff at Springer for their support and enthusiasm for the production of this book.

Most of the uninterrupted work was done at night well into the early hours of the morning after clinics and surgery and over the weekends. Therefore, I am also appreciative of my parents, family, especially my brother Dr. Seyed Behzad Mostofi, and friends who understood the value of this to me and forgave me for being constantly absent from social gatherings and adjusted themselves to my difficult hours of solitary work. I am grateful to them all. I accept responsibility for any shortcomings in this book and can assure you that corrections will be gladly made in the next edition.

Contents

Chapter 1
Spine

Cervical Spine

Injuries to the Occiput C1-C2 Complex

Anderson and Montisano Classification of Occipital
Condyle Fractures

Type I: Impaction of condyle.
Type II: Associated with basilar or skull fractures.
Type III: Condylar avulsion.

Atlanto-Occipital Dislocation (Craniovertebral Dissociation)

Classified Based on Position of the Occiput in Relation to C1

Type I: Occipital condyles anterior to the atlas; most common.
Type II: Condyles longitudinally result of pure distraction.
Type III: Occipital condyles posterior to the atlas.

S.B. Mostofi, *Fracture Classifications in Clinical Practice*
Second Edition, DOI 10.1007/978-1-4471-4420-5_1,
© Springer-Verlag London 2012

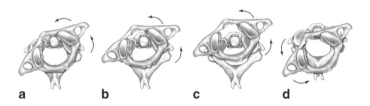

a   **b**   **c**   **d**

FIGURE 1.1 Fielding classification of atlantoaxial rotatory subluxation and dislocation [1]

Atlas Fractures

Levine and Edwards Classification

1. Burst fracture (Jefferson fracture). Axial load injury resulting in four fractures; two in posterior arch, two in anterior arch.
2. Posterior arch fractures. Hyperextension injury; associated with odontoid and axis fractures.
3. Comminuted fractures. Axial load and lateral bending injury; associated with high non-union rate and poor clinical result.
4. Anterior arch fractures. Hyperextension injury.
5. Lateral mass fractures. Axial load and lateral bending injury.
6. Transverse process fracture. Avulsion injury.
7. Inferior tubercle fracture. Avulsion of the longus colli muscle.

Atlantoaxial Rotary Subluxation and Dislocation

Fielding Classification (Fig. 1.1)

Type I: Simple rotatory displacement without anterior shift. Odontoid acts as a pivot point; Transverse ligament intact.

Type II: Rotatory displacement with anterior displacement of 3.5 mm. Opposite facet acts as a pivot; transverse ligament insufficient.

Type III: Rotatory displacement with anterior displacement of more than 5 mm. Both joints anteriorly subluxed. Transverse and alar ligaments incompetent.

Type IV: Rare; both joints posteriorly subluxed.

Type V: (Levine and Edwards) frank dislocation; extremely rare.

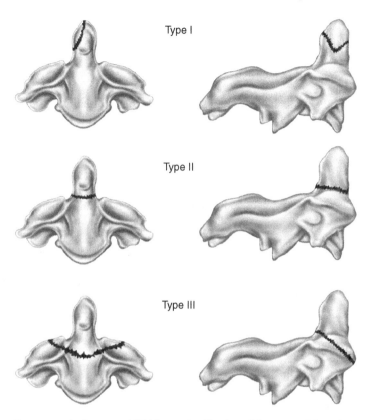

FIGURE 1.2 Anderson and D'Alonzo classification of fractures of the odontoid process (Dens) [2]

Fractures of the Odontoid Process (Dens)

Anderson and D'Alonzo Classification (Fig. 1.2)

Type I: Oblique avulsion fracture of the apex (5 %).
Type II: Fracture at the junction of the body and the neck; high non-union rate (60 %).
Type III: Fracture extends into the body of C-2 and may involve the lateral facets (30 %).

Traumatic Spondylolisthesis of Axis (Hangman's Fracture)

Levine and Edwards Classification (Fig. 1.3)

Type I: Minimally displaced, no angulation; translation <3 mm; stable.

Type II: Significant angulation at C2-3; translation >3 mm; unstable; C2-3 disc disrupted. Subclassified into flexion, extension, and listhetic types.

> Type IIA: Avulsion of entire C2-3 intervertebral disc in flexion, leaving the anterior longitudinal ligament intact. Results in severe angulation. No translation; unstable; due to flexion-distraction injury.

Type III: Rare; results from initial anterior facet dislocation of C-2 on C-3 followed by extension injury fracturing the neural arch. Results in severe angulation and translation with unilateral or bilateral facet dislocation of C2-3; unstable.

Injuries to C3-7

Allen Classification

1. Compressive flexion (shear mechanism resulting in "teardrop" fractures)

    Stage I: Blunting of anterior body; posterior element intact.

    Stage II: "Beaking" of the anterior body; loss of anterior vertebral height.

    Stage III: Fracture line passing from anterior body through the inferior subchondral plate.

    Stage IV: Inferoposterior margin displaced <3 mm into the spinal canal.

    Stage V: Teardrop fracture; inferoposterior margin >3 mm into the spinal canal; posterior ligaments and the posterior longitudinal ligament have failed.

2. Vertical compression (burst fractures)

    Stage I: Fracture through superior or inferior endplate with no displacement.

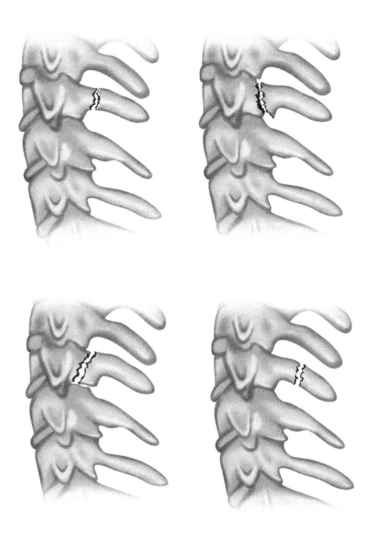

FIGURE 1.3 Levine and Edwards classification of traumatic spondylolisthesis of axis: Type I (*top left*), Type II (*top right*), Type IIA (*bottom left*), Type III (*bottom right*) [3]

Stage II: Fracture through both endplates with minimal displacement.

Stage III: Burst fracture; displacement of fragments peripherally and into the neural canal.

3. Distractive flexion (dislocations)

Stage I: Failure of the posterior ligaments, divergence of spinous processes, and facet subluxation.

Stage II: Unilateral facet dislocation; displacement is always <50 %.

Stage III: Bilateral facet dislocation; displacement >50 %.

Stage IV: Bilateral facet dislocation with 100 % translation.

4. Compressive extension

Stage I: Unilateral vertebral arch fracture.

Stage II: Bilaminar fracture without other tissue failure.

Stage III: Bilateral vertebral arch fracture with fracture of the articular processes, pedicles, and lamina without vertebral body displacement.

Stage IV: Bilateral vertebral arch fracture with full vertebral body displacement anteriorly; ligamentous failure at the posterosuperior and anteroinferior margins.

5. Distractive extension

Stage I: Failure of anterior ligamentous complex or transverse fracture of the body; widening of the disc space and no posterior displacement.

Stage II: Failure of posterior ligament complex with displacement of the vertebral body into the canal.

6. Lateral flexion

Stage I: Asymmetric unilateral compression fracture of the vertebral body plus a vertebral arch fracture on the ipsilateral side without displacement.

Stage II: Displacement of the arch on the anteroposterior view or failure of the ligaments on the contralateral side with articular process separation.

Orthopedic Trauma Association (OTA) Classification of Cervical Spine Injuries

Type A: Compression injuries of the body (compressive forces)
Type A1: Impaction fractures
Type A2: Split fractures
Type A3: Burst fractures

Type B: Distraction injuries of the anterior and posterior elements (tensile forces)

 Type B2: Posterior disruption predominantly osseous (flexion-distraction injury)

 Type B3: Anterior disruption through the disk (hyperextension-shear injury)

Type C: Multidirectional injuries with translation affecting the anterior and posterior elements (axial torque causing rotation injuries)

 Type C1: Rotational wedge, split, and burst fractures

 Type C2: Flexion subluxation with rotation

 Type C3: Rotational shear injuries (Holdsworth slice rotation fracture)

Thoracolumbar Spine Fractures

McAfee Classification

Classification is based on the failure mode of the middle osteoligamentous complex (posterior longitudinal ligament, posterior half of the vertebral body, and posterior annulus fibrosus).
The six injury patterns are the following:

1. Wedge-compression fracture
2. Stable burst fracture
3. Unstable burst fracture
4. Chance fracture
5. Flexion-distraction injury
6. Translational injuries

Denis Classification

The three-column model according to Denis (Fig. 1.4):

Anterior column
 Anterior longitudinal ligament
 Anterior half of vertebral body
 Anterior portion of annulus fibrosis
Middle column
 Posterior longitudinal ligament
 Posterior half of vertebral body
 Posterior aspect of annulus fibrosis

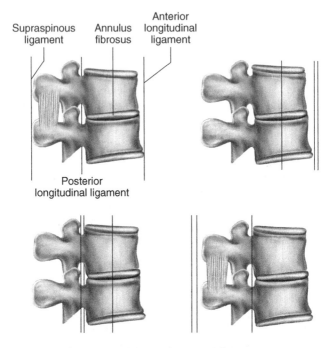

FIGURE 1.4 Denis' concept of three-column model

Posterior column
    Neural arch
    Ligamentum flavum
    Facet capsule
    Interspinus ligament

TABLE 1.1 Pattern of failure

Type	Column		
	Anterior	**Middle**	**Posterior**
1. Compression	Compression	None	None/distraction
2. Burst	Compression	Compression	None/splaying of pedicles
3. Flexion-distraction	None/ distraction	Distraction	Distraction
4. Flexion-dislocation	Compression/ rotation/shear	Compression/ rotation/shear	Compression/ rotation/shear

Based on three-column model, classifying fractures according to the mechanism of injury and the resulting fracture pattern into (Table 1.1):

1. Compression
2. Burst
3. Flexion-distraction
4. Fracture-dislocation

1. *Compression Fractures*
Four subtypes described on the basis of endplate involvement are as follows:
Type A: Fracture of both endplates
Type B: Fractures of the superior endplate
Type C: Fractures of the inferior endplate
Type D: Both endplates intact

2. *Burst Fractures* (Fig. 1.5)
Type A: Fractures of both endplates
Type B: Fracture of the superior endplate
Type C: Fracture of the inferior endplate
Type D: Burst rotation
Type E: Burst lateral flexion

3. *Flexion-Distraction Injuries (Chance Fractures, Seat Belt-Type Injuries)*
Type A: One-level bony injury
Type B: One-level ligamentous
Type C: Two-level injury through bony middle column
Type D: Two-level injury through ligamentous middle column

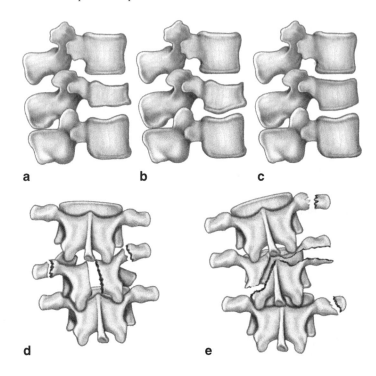

FIGURE 1.5 Burst thoracolumbar spine fractures

4. *Fracture Dislocations*

Type A: Flexion-rotation. Posterior and middle column fail in tension and rotation; anterior column fails in compression and rotation; 75 % have neurological deficits, 52 % of these are complete lesions.

Type B: Shear. Shear failure of all three columns, most commonly in the postero-anterior direction; all cases with complete neurological deficits.

Type C: Flexion-distraction. Tension failure of posterior and middle columns, with anterior tear of annulus fibrosus and stripping of the anterior longitudinal ligament; 75 % with neurological deficits (all incomplete).

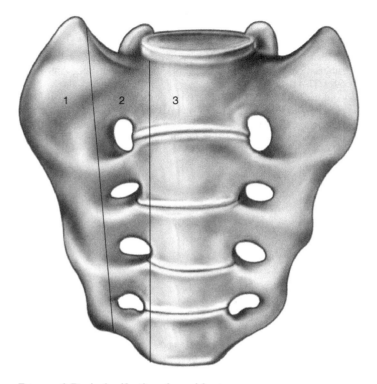

FIGURE 1.6 Denis classification of sacral fractures

Sacral Fractures (Fig. 1.6)

Denis Classification

Zone 1: The region of the ala
Zone 2: The region of the sacral foramina
Zone 3: The region of central sacral canal

References

1. Fielding WJ, Hawkins RJ. Atlanto-axial rotatory fixation (fixed rotatory subluxation of the atlantoaxial joint). J Bone Joint Surg Am. 1977; 59-A:37–44.
2. Anderson LD, Alonzo RT. Fractures of the odontoid process of the axis. J Bone Joint Surg Am. 1974;56A:1663–74.
3. Levine AM, Edwards CC. The management of traumatic spondylolisthesis of the axis. J Bone Joint Surg Am. 1985;67A:217–26.

Chapter 2
Shoulder and Upper Limb

Clavicle

Craig Classification

Group I: Fracture of the middle third
Group II: Fracture of the distal third. Subclassified according to the location of coracoclavicular ligaments relative to the fracture as follows:

    Type I: Minimal displacement—interligamentous fracture between conoid and trapezoid or between the coracoclavicular and acromio-cavicular ligaments

    Type II: Displaced secondary to a fracture medial to the coracoclavicular ligaments—higher incidence of non-union

        IIA: Conoid and trapezoid attached to the distal segment (Fig. 2.1)

        IIB: Conoid torn, trapezoid attached to the distal segment (Fig. 2.2)

    Type III: Fracture of the articular surface of the acromioclavicular joint with no ligamentous injury—may be confused with first-degree acromioclavicular joint separation

Group III: Fracture of the proximal third

    Type I: Minimal displacement
    Type II: Significant displaced (ligamentous rupture)
    Type III: Intraarticular
    Type IV: Epiphyseal separation
    Type V: Comminuted

S.B. Mostofi, *Fracture Classifications in Clinical Practice*   13
Second Edition, DOI 10.1007/978-1-4471-4420-5_2,
© Springer-Verlag London 2012

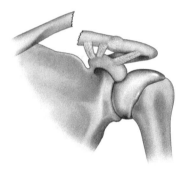

FIGURE 2.1 Type IIA clavicular fracture according to Craig classification [1]

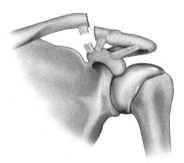

FIGURE 2.2 Type IIB clavicular fracture according to Craig classification [1]

Acromioclavicular Joint

Rockwood Classification (Fig. 2.3)

Type I: Sprain of the AC ligament
           AC joint tenderness, minimal pain with arm motion, no
           pain in coracoclavicular interspaces.
           No abnormality on radiographs.
Type II: AC ligament tear with joint disruption, coracoclavicular
           ligaments sprained. Distal clavicle is slightly superior to

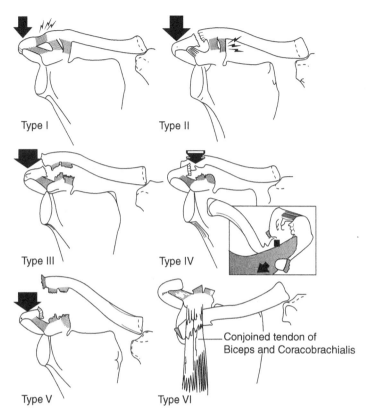

FIGURE 2.3 Types I–VI of the Rockwood classification for acromioclavicular joints [2]

acromion and mobile to palpation; tenderness is found in the coracoclavicular space.

Radiographs demonstrate slight elevation of the distal end of the clavicle and AC joint widening. Stress films show the coracoclavicular ligaments are sprained but integrity is maintained.

Type III: AC and coracoclavicular ligaments torn with AC joint dislocation; deltoid and trapezius muscles usually detached from the distal clavicle.

The upper extremity and distal fragment are depressed, and the distal end of the proximal fragment may tent the skin. The AC joint is tender, coracoclavicular widening is evident.

Radiographs demonstrate the distal clavicle superior to the medial border of the acromion; stress views reveal a widened coracoclavicular interspace 25–100 % greater than the normal side.

Type IV: Type III with the distal clavicle displaced posteriorly into or through the trapezius.

Clinically, more pain exists than in type III; the distal clavicle is displaced posteriorly away from the clavicle.

Axillary radiograph or computed tomography demonstrates posterior displacement of the distal clavicle.

Type V: Type III with the distal clavicle grossly and severely displaced superiorly.

This type is typically associated with tenting of the skin. Radiographs demonstrate the coracoclavicular interspace to be 100–300 % greater than the normal side.

Type VI: AC dislocated, with the clavicle displaced inferior to the acromion or the coracoid; the coracoclavicular interspace is decreased compared with normal.

The deltoid and trapezius muscles are detached from the distal clavicle.

The mechanism of injury is usually a severe direct force onto the superior surface of the distal clavicle, with abduction of the arm and scapula retraction.

Clinically, the shoulder has a flat appearance with a prominent acromion; associated clavicle and upper rib fractures and brachial plexus injuries are due to high-energy trauma.

Radiographs demonstrate one of two types of inferior dislocation: subacromial or subcoracoid.

Sternoclavicular Joint

Anatomic Classification

Anterior dislocation—more common
Posterior dislocation

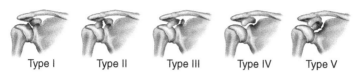

FIGURE 2.4 Types I–V of the Eyres and Brooks classification for coracoid fractures [3]

Etiologic Classification

Sprain or subluxation
  Mild: joint stable, ligamentous integrity maintained
  Moderate: subluxation, with partial ligamentous disruption
  Severe: unstable joint, with complete ligamentous compromise

Scapula

Zdravkovic and Damholt Classification

Type I: Scapula body
Type II: Apophyseal fractures, including the acromion and coracoid
Type III: Fractures of the superolateral angle, including the scapular neck and glenoid

Coracoid Fractures

Eyres and Brooks Classification (Fig. 2.4)

Type I: Coracoid tip or epiphyseal fracture
Type II: Mid process
Type III: Basal fracture
Type IV: Involvement of superior body of scapula
Type V: Extension into the glenoid fossa

The suffix of A or B can be used to record the presence of absence of damage to the clavicle or its ligamentous connection to the scapula.

Intraarticular Glenoid Fractures

Ideberg Classification (Fig. 2.5)

Type I: Avulsion fracture of the anterior margin
Type IIA: Transverse fracture through the glenoid fossa exiting inferiorly
Type IIB: Oblique fracture through the glenoid fossa exiting inferiorly
Type III: Oblique fracture through the glenoid exiting superiorly; often associated with an acromioclavicular joint injury
Type IV: Transverse fracture exiting through the medial border of the scapula
Type V: Combination of a type II and type IV pattern
Type VI: Sever continuation of glenoid surface (GOSS)

Anterior Glenohumeral Dislocation

Classification

Degree of instability
Dislocation/subluxation
Chronology/type
    Congenital
    Acute versus chronic
    Locked (fixed)
    Recurrent
Force
    Atraumatic
    Traumatic
Patient contribution
Voluntary/involuntary
Direction
    Subcoracoid
    Subglenoid
    Intrathoracic

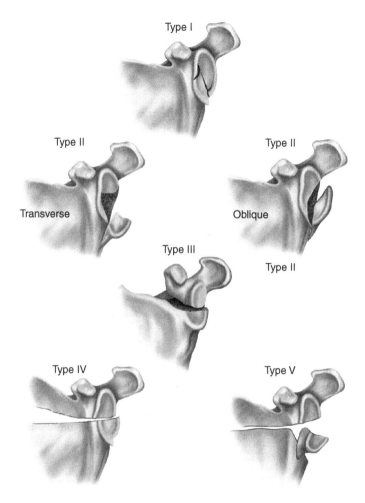

FIGURE 2.5 Ideberg classification of intraarticular glenoid fractures [4]

Posterior Glenohumeral Dislocation

Anatomic Classification

Subacromial (98 %). Articular surface directed posteriorly; the lesser tuberosity typically occupies the glenoid fossa; often associated with an impaction fracture on the anterior humeral head.
Subglenoid (very rare). Humeral head posterior and inferior to the glenoid
Subspinous (very rare). Humeral head medial to the acromion and inferior to the spine of the Scapula.

Inferior Glenohumeral Dislocation (Luxatio Erecta)

Superior Glenohumeral Dislocation

Proximal Humerus

Neer Classification (Fig. 2.6)

- The four parts are the greater and lesser tuberosities, the shaft, and the humeral head.
- A part is displaced if >1 cm of displacement or >45° of angulation is seen.
- At least two views of the proximal humerus (anteroposterior and scapular Y views) must be obtained; additionally, the axillary view is very helpful for ruling out dislocation.

Humeral Shaft

Descriptive Classification

Open/closed
Location: proximal third, middle third, distal third
Degree: incomplete, complete
Direction and character: transverse, oblique, spiral, segmental, comminuted
Intrinsic condition of the bone
Articular extension

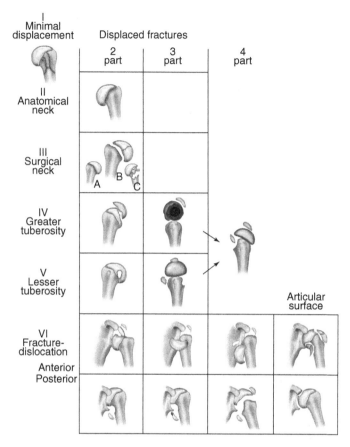

FIGURE 2.6 Neer classification of fractures to the proximal humerus [5]

AO Classification of Humeral Diaphyseal Fractures
(Fig. 2.7)

Type A: Simple fracture
            A1: Spiral
            A2: Oblique ($>30°$)
            A3: Transverse ($<30°$)
Type B: Wedge fracture
            B1: Spiral wedge
            B2: Bending wedge
            B3: Fragmented wedge
Type C: Complex fracture
            C1: Spiral
            C2: Segmented
            C3: Irregular (significant comminution)

Distal Humerus

Descriptive

Supracondylar Fractures
    Extension Type
    Flexion Type
Transcondylar Fractures
    Fracture passes through both condyles and is within the joint
    capsule.
Condylar Fracture
    Medial
    Lateral

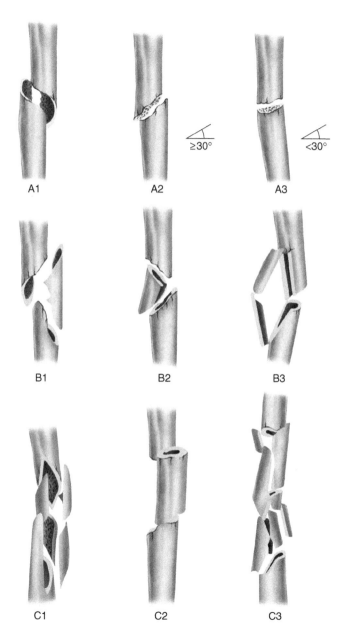

≥30°

<30°

A1

A2

A3

B1

B2

B3

C1

C2

C3

FIGURE 2.7 AO classification of humeral diaphyseal fractures

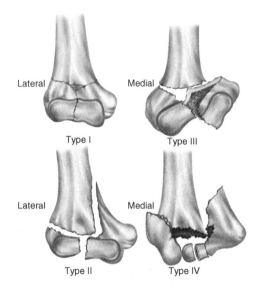

FIGURE 2.8 *Type I*, *Type II*, *Type III*, and *Type IV* intercondylar fractures [6]

Intercondylar Fractures

Riseborough and Radin Classification (Fig. 2.8)

Type I: Nondisplaced
Type II: Slight displacement with no rotation between the condy-
            lar fragments in the frontal plane
Type III: Displacement with rotation
Type IV: Severe comminution of the articular surface

Condylar Fractures

Milch Classification (Fig. 2.9)

Two types for medial and lateral; the key is the lateral trochlear ridge.

Type I: Lateral trochlear ridge is left intact
Type II: Lateral trochlear ridge is part of the condylar fragment
            (medial or lateral)

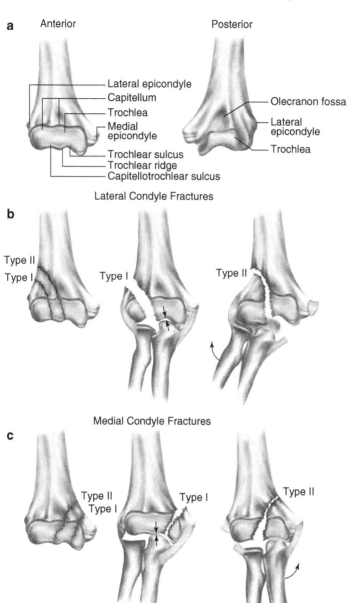

FIGURE 2.9 Milch classification of condylar fractures [7]

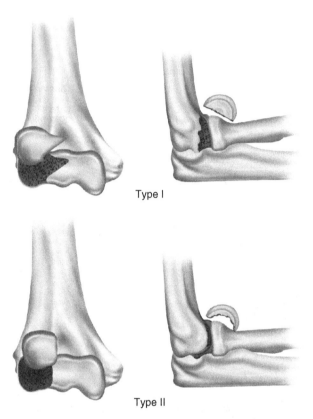

Type I

Type II

FIGURE 2.10 Types I and II classification of capitellum fractures [2, 8–11]

Capitellum Fractures

Classification (Fig. 2.10)

Type I: Hahn-Steinthal fragment. Large osseous component of
             capitellum, sometimes with trochlear involvement
Type II: Kocher-Lorenz fragment. Articular cartilage with minimal
             subchondral bone attached :"uncapping of the condyle"
Type III: Markedly comminuted

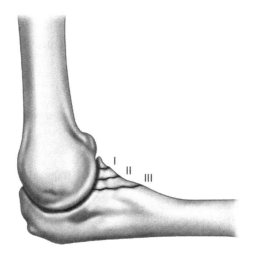

FIGURE 2.11 Regan and Morrey classification of coronoid process fractures [12]

Coronoid Process Fracture

Regan and Morrey Classification (Fig. 2.11)

Type I: Fracture avulsion just the tip of the coronoid
Type II: Those that involve less than 50 % of coronoid either as single fracture or multiple fragments
Type III: Those involve >50 % of coronoid
            Subdivision into A: Without elbow dislocation
                            B: With elbow dislocation

Olecranon

The Mayo Classification of Olecranon Fractures (Fig. 2.12)

Type I: Nondisplaced or minimally displaced
        IA: Noncomminuted
        IB: Comminuted
Type II: Displacement of proximal fragment without elbow instability
        IIA: Noncomminuted
        IIB: Comminuted
Type III: Displaced fracture of proximal fragment with elbow instability
        IIIA: Noncomminuted
        IIIB: Comminuted

Type I Undisplaced

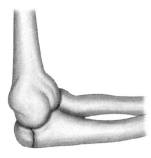 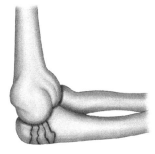

Type II Displaced – stable

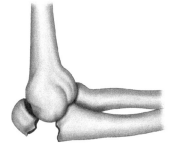 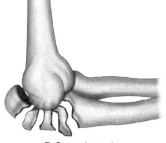

A-Noncomminuted   B-Comminuted

Type III Unstable

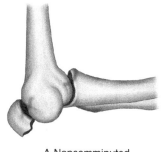 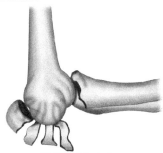

A-Noncomminuted   B-Comminuted

FIGURE 2.12 Mayo Classification

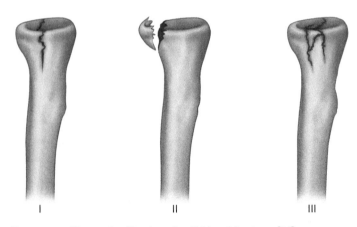

FIGURE 2.13 Mason classification of radial head fractures [14]

Radial Head

Mason Classification (Fig. 2.13)

Type I: Nondisplaced marginal fractures
Type II: Marginal fractures with displacement (impaction, depression, angulation)
Type III: Comminuted fractures involving the entire head
Type IV: Associated with dislocation of the elbow (Johnston)

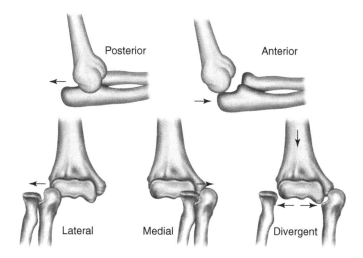

FIGURE 2.14 Classification of elbow dislocation

Elbow Dislocation

Classification (Fig. 2.14)

Chronology: Acute, chronic (unreduced), recurrent
Descriptive: Based on relationship of radius/ulna to the distal humerus, as follows:

- Posterior
    Posterolateral: >90 % dislocations
    Posteromedial
- Anterior
- Lateral
- Medial
- Divergent (rare)

Anterior-posterior type (ulna posterior, radial head anterior).
Mediolateral (transverse) type (distal humerus wedged between radius lateral and ulna medial).

Forearm

Descriptive Classification

- Closed versus open
- Location
- Comminuted, segmental, or multifragmented
- Displacement
- Angulation
- Rotational alignment

Monteggia Fractures (Fig. 2.15)

Fracture of the shaft of the ulna with associated dislocation of the radial head.

Bado Classification

Type I: Anterior dislocation of the radial head with fracture of the ulnar diaphysis at any level with anterior angulation

Type II: Posterior/posterolateral dislocation of the radial head with fracture of the ulnar diaphysis with posterior angulation

Type III: Lateral/anterolateral dislocation of the radial head with fracture of the ulnar metaphysic

Type IV: Anterior dislocation of the radial head with fractures of both the radius and ulna within proximal third at the same level

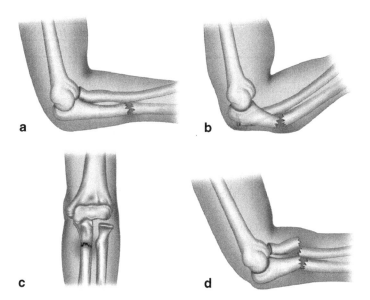

FIGURE 2.15 Monteggia fractures [15]

TABLE 2.1 Frykman classification of distal radius

| Fracture | Distal ulnar fracture | |
	Absent	Present
Extraarticular	I	II
Intraarticular involving radiocarpal joint	III	IV
Intraarticular involving distal radioulnar joint	V	VI
Intraarticular involving radiocarpal and distal radioulnar joint	VII	VIII

Distal Radius (Table 2.1 and Fig. 2.16)

Descriptive Classification

- Open/closed
- Displacement
- Angulation
- Comminution
- Loss of radial length
- Intraarticular involvement

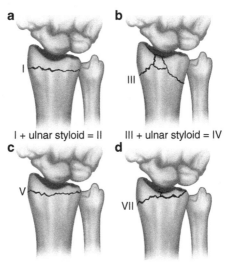

FIGURE 2.16 Fractures of the distal radius [21]

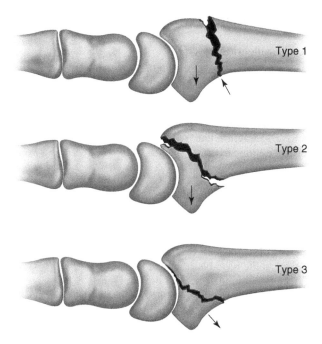

FIGURE 2.17 Modified Thomas' classification [16]

Smith Fracture

Modified Thomas' Classification (Fig. 2.17)

Type I: Extraarticular
Type II: Fracture line crosses into the dorsal articular surface
Type III: Fracture line enters the carpal joint (Volar Barton)

Scaphoid Fractures

Russe Classification

1. Horizontal oblique
   Distal third
   Middle third (waist)
   Proximal third
2. Transverse fracture line
3. Vertical oblique fracture line

Herbert and Fisher Classification (Fig. 2.18)

Type A: Acute stable fractures
          A1: Fracture of tubercle
          A2: Undisplaced "crack" fracture of the waist
Type B: Acute unstable fractures
          B1: Oblique fractures of distal third
          B2: Displaced or mobile fracture of the waist
          B3: Proximal pole fractures
          B4: Fracture dislocation of carpus
          B5: Comminuted fractures
Type C: Delayed union
Type D: Established nonunion
          D1: Fibrous nonunion
          D2: Sclerotic nonunion (Pseudoarthrosis)

Note that stable indicates nondisplaced fractures with no stepoff in any plane; unstable indicates displacement with 1 mm or more step-off with scapholunate angulation >60° or lunatocapitate angulation >15°.

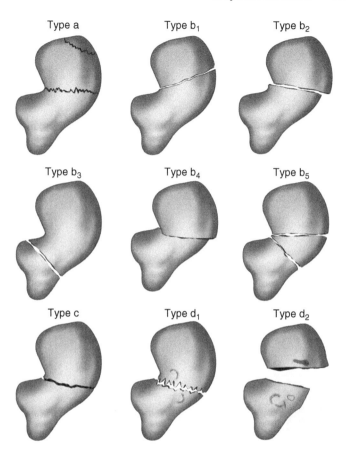

FIGURE 2.18 Herbert and Fisher classification [17]

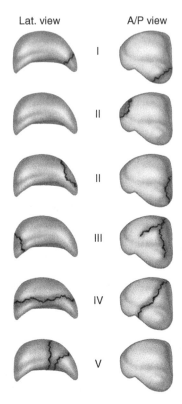

FIGURE 2.19 Teisen and Hjarbaek classification. Left: lateral view; right: AP view [18]

Lunate Fractures

Teisen and Hjarkbaek Classification (Fig. 2.19)

Group I: Fracture volar pole, possibly affecting the volar nutrient artery

Group II: Chip fracture which does not affect the main blood supply

Group III: Fracture of dorsal pole of the Lunate possibly affecting the blood supply

Group IV: Sagittal fracture through the body of lunate

Group V: Transverse fractures through the body of the lunate

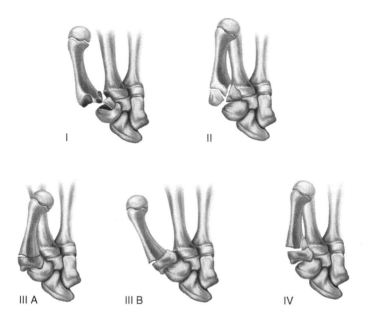

FIGURE 2.20 Intraarticular fractures of the thumb [19]

Thumb

Intraarticular Fractures (Fig. 2.20)

Type I: Bennett fracture—fracture line separates major part of
           metacarpal from volar lip fragment, producing a disrup-
           tion of the first carpometacarpal joint; first metacarpal is
           pulled proximally by the abductor pollicis longus.

Type II: Rolando fracture—requires greater force than a Bennett
           fracture; presently used to describe a comminuted
           Bennett fracture, a "Y" or "T" fracture, or a fracture with
           dorsal and palmar fragments.

Extraarticular Fractures

Type IIIA: Transverse fracture
Type IIIB: Oblique fracture
Type IV: Epiphyseal injuries seen in children

Distal Phalanx Fractures

Kaplan Classification

Type I: Longitudinal split
Type II: Comminuted tuft
Type III: Transverse fracture

Mallet Fracture

Wehbe and Schnider Classification (Fig. 2.21)

Type I: Mallet fractures including bone injuries of varying extend without subluxation of distal interphalangyal joint
Type II: Fractures are associated with subluxation distal interphalangyal joint
Type III: Epiphyseal and physeal injuries
             Each type then divided into three subtypes:
             A: Fracture fragment involving less than 1/3 of articular surface of distal phalanx
             B: Fracture fragment involving 1/3–2/3 of articular surface
             C: Fragment that involves more than 2/3 of articular surface

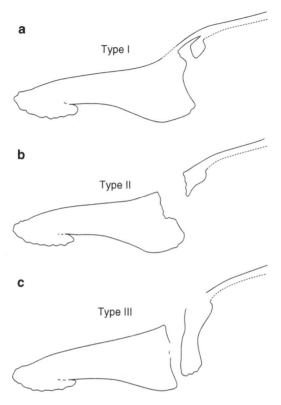

a

Type I

b

Type II

c

Type III

FIGURE 2.21 Wehbe and Schneider classification [20]

References

1. Craig EV. Fractures of the clavicle. In: Rockwood CA, Matsen FA, editors. The shoulder. Philadelphia: Saunders; 1990.
2. Heckman JD, Bucholz RW, editors. Rockwood, Green and Wilkins' fractures in adults. Philadelphia: Lippincott Williams & Wilkins; 2001.
3. Eyre KS, Brook A, Stanley D. Fractures of coracoid process. J Bone Joint Surg Br. 1995;77B:425–8.
4. Ideberg R. Fractures of the scapula involving the glenoid fossa. In: Batemans JE, Welsh RP, editors. The surgery of the shoulder. Philadelphia: Decker; 1984. p. 63–6.
5. Neer CS. Displaced proximal humeral fractures: I. Classification and evaluation. J Bone Joint Surg Am. 1970;52A:1077–89.
6. Riseborough EJ, Radin EL. Intercondylar T fractures of the humerus in the adult. A comparison of operative and non operative treatment in twenty-nine cases. J Bone Joint Surg Am. 1969;51A: 130–41.
7. Milch H. Fractures and fracture-dislocations of the humeral condyles. J Trauma. 1964;4:592–607.
8. Hahn NF. Fall von cine besonderes varietat der frakturen des ellenbogens. Z Wundarzte Geburtshilfe. 1853;6:185–9.
9. Steinthal D. Die isolierte fraktur der eminentia capitata in ellenbogengelenk. Zentralbl Chir. 1898;15:17–20.
10. Kocher T. Beitrage zur Kenntniss Einiger Tisch Wichtiger Frakturformen. Basel, Sallman, 1896:585–591
11. Lorenz H. Zur kenntniss der fractura humeri (eminentiae capitatae). Dtsch Z Chir. 1905;78:531–45.
12. Regan W, Morrey B. Fracture of coronoid process of the ulna. J Bone Joint Surg Am. 1989;71-A:1348–54.
13. Morrey BF. Current concepts in the treatment of fractures of the radial head, the olecranon, and the coronoid. J Bone Joint Surg Am. 1995;77:316–27.
14. Mason ML. Some observations on fractures of the head of the radius with a review of one hundred cases. Br J Surg. 1954;42:123–32.
15. Bado JL. The monteggia lesion. Clin Orthop. 1967;50:70–86.
16. Thomas FB. Reduction of Smith's fracture. J Bone Joint Surg. 1957;39B:463–70.
17. Herbert T, Fisher W. Management of the fractured scaphoid using a new bone screw. J Bone Joint Surg. 1984;66B:114–23.
18. Teisen H, Hjarbaek J. Classification of fresh fractures. J Hand Surg Br. 1988;13(B):458–62.
19. Green DP, O'Brien ET. Fractures of the thumb metacarpal. South Med J. 1972;65:807.

20. Wehbe MA, Schneider LH. Mallet fractures. J Bone Joint Surg Am. 1984;66-A:658–69.
21. Frykman G. Fracture of the distal radius including sequelae—shoulder-hand-finger syndrome, disturbance in the distal radio-ulnar joint, and impairment of nerve function: a clinical and experimental study. Acta Orthop Scand. 1967;108(Suppl):1–153.

Chapter 3
Pelvis and Lower Limb

Pelvis

Young and Burgess Classification (Fig. 3.1)

1. Lateral compression
2. Anteroposterior compression
3. Vertical shear
4. Combined mechanical

Description:

1. Lateral compression (LC): Transverse fractures of the pubic rami, ipsilateral or contralateral to posterior injury.
   Type I: Sacral compression on the side of impact
   Type II: Posterior iliac wing fracture (crescent) on the side of impact
   Type III: LC-I or LC-II injury on the side of impact; contralateral open book injury

2. Anteroposterior compression: symphyseal diastasis; or longitudinal rami fractures
   Type I: <2.5 cm of symphyseal diastasis; vertical fractures of one or both pubic rami intact posterior ligaments.
   Type II: <2.5 cm of symphyseal diastasis; widening of sacroiliac joint due to anterior sacroiliac ligament disruption; disruption of the sacrotuberous, sacrospinous, and symphyseal ligaments with intact posterior sacroiliac ligaments result in "open book" injury with internal and external rotational instability; vertical stability is maintained.

S.B. Mostofi, *Fracture Classifications in Clinical Practice*
Second Edition, DOI 10.1007/978-1-4471-4420-5_3,
© Springer-Verlag London 2012

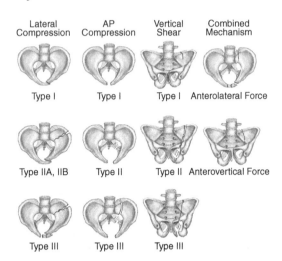

FIGURE 3.1 Young and Burgess classification of pelvic ring fractures [1]

    Type III: Complete disruption of the symphysis, sacrotuberous, sacrospinous, and sacroiliac ligaments resulting in extreme rotational instability and lateral displacement; no cephaloposterior displacement; completely unstable with the highest rate of associated neurovascular injuries and blood loss.

3. Vertical shear: symphyseal diastasis or vertical displaced anterior and posterior usually through the SI joint, occasionally through the iliac wing or sacrum.
4. Combined mechanical: combination of injuries often due to crush mechanisms; most common is vertical shear and lateral compression.

Tile Classification

Type A: Stable
            A1: Fractures of the pelvis not involving the ring; avulsion injuries
            A2: Stable, minimally displaced fractures of the ring

Type B: Rotationally unstable, vertically stable
            B1: Open-book
            B2: Lateral compression; ipsilateral
            B3: Lateral compression; contralateral (bucket handle)

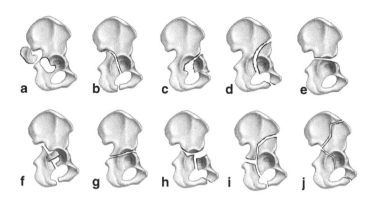

FIGURE 3.2 Fractures of the acetabulum [2]

Type C: Rotationally and vertically unstable
      C1:   Unilateral
      C2:   Bilateral; one side rotationally unstable, with contralateral side vertically unstable
      C3:   Associated acetabular fracture

Acetabulum

Judet-Letournel Classification (Fig. 3.2)

Elementary patterns:
1. Posterior wall
2. Posterior column
3. Anterior wall
4. Anterior column
5. Transverse

Associated patterns:
1. T-shaped
2. Posterior column and posterior wall
3. Transverse and posterior wall
4. Anterior column:
   Posterior
   Hemitransverse
5. Both columns

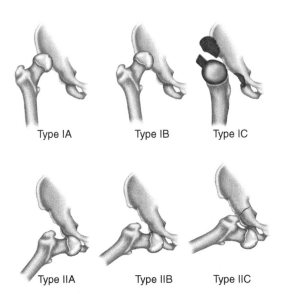

Type IA   Type IB   Type IC

Type IIA   Type IIB   Type IIC

FIGURE 3.3 Epstein classification of anterior dislocations of the hip

Hip Dislocations

Anterior Dislocations

Inferior (obturator) dislocation
Superior (iliac or pubic) dislocation

Epstein Classification of Anterior Dislocations of the Hip
(Fig. 3.3)

Type I: Superior dislocations, including pubic and subspinous
           IA: No associated fractures
           IB: Associated fracture or impaction of the femoral head
           IC: Associated fracture of the acetabulum

Type II: Inferior dislocations, including obturator and perineal
           IIA: No associated fractures
           IIB: Associated fractures or impaction of the femoral
                head/neck
           IIC: Associated fracture of the acetabulum

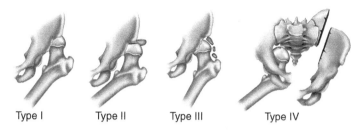

Type I   Type II   Type III   Type IV

FIGURE 3.4 Thompson and Epstein classification of posterior dislocations of the hip

Posterior Dislocation

Thompson and Epstein Classification of Posterior Dislocations of the Hip (Fig. 3.4)

Type I: Dislocation with or without an insignificant posterior wall fragment
Type II: Dislocation associated with a single large posterior wall fragment
Type III: Dislocation with a comminuted posterior wall fragment
Type IV: Dislocation with fracture of the acetabular floor
Type V: Dislocation with fracture of the femoral head

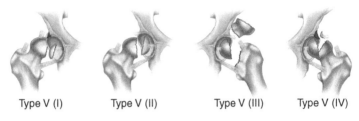

| Type V (I) | Type V (II) | Type V (III) | Type V (IV) |

FIGURE 3.5 Pipkin classification of femoral head fractures [3]

Femoral Head

The Thompson & Epstein type V fracture dislocation has been subclassified into four types:

Pipkin Subclassification (Fig. 3.5)

Type I: Posterior hip dislocation with fracture of the femoral head inferior to the fovea centralis
Type II: Posterior hip dislocation with fracture of the femoral head superior to the fovea centralis
Type III: Type II injury or I associated with fracture of the femoral neck
Type IV: Type II injury or I associated with fracture of the acetabular rim

Stewart-Milford Classification of Hip Dislocation

Grade I: Dislocation without an associated fracture or only small bony avulsion of the acetabular rim
Grade II: Posterior rim fracture with a stable hip after reduction
Grade III: Posterior rim fracture with an unstable hip
Grade IV: Dislocation with associated fracture of the femoral head or neck

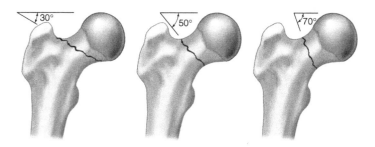

FIGURE 3.6 Pauwels classification of femoral neck fractures

Femoral Neck Fractures

Classification by Anatomic Location

- Subcapital
- Transcervical
- Basicervical

Pauwels Classification (Fig. 3.6)

Based on angle of fracture from horizontal plane

Type I: 30°
Type II: 50°
Type III: 70°

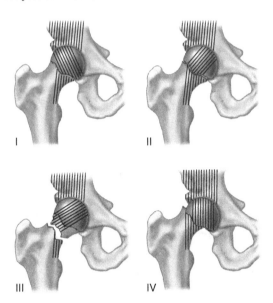

FIGURE 3.7 Garden classification of femoral neck fractures [4]

Garden Classification (Fig. 3.7)

Based on degree of valgus displacement.

Stage I: Incomplete/impacted
Stage II: Complete nondisplaced on anteroposterior and lateral views
Stage III: Complete with partial displacement; trabecular pattern of the femoral head does not line up with that of the acetabulum
Stage IV: Completely displaced; trabecular pattern of the head assumes a parallel orientation with that of the acetabulum

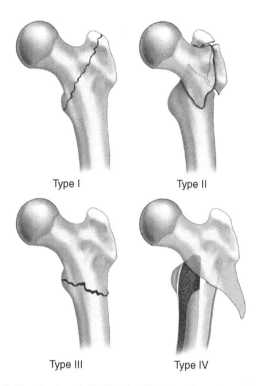

Type I

Type II

Type III

Type IV

FIGURE 3.8 The Boyd and Griffin classification of trochanteric fractures: Type I (*top left*), Type II (*top right*), Type III (*bottom left*), Type IV (*bottom right*) [5]

Intertrochanteric Fractures

Boyd and Griffin Classification (Fig. 3.8)

Type I: A single fracture along the intertrochanteric line, stable and easily reducible

Type II: Major fracture line along the intertrochanteric line with comminution in the coronal plane

Type III: Fracture at the level of the lesser trochanter with variable comminution and extension into the subtrochanteric region (reverse obliquity)

Type IV: Fracture extending into the proximal femoral shaft in at least two planes

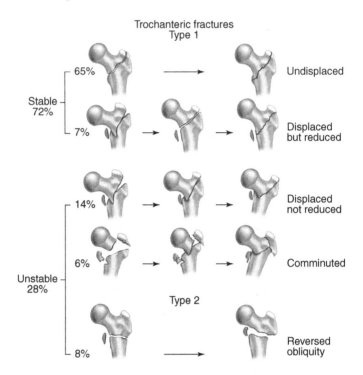

FIGURE 3.9 Trochanteric fractures [6]

Evans Classification (Fig. 3.9)

Type I:

Stable:
- Undisplaced fractures
- Displaced but after reduction overlap of the medial cortical buttress make the fracture stable

Unstable:
- Displaced and the medial cortical buttress is not restored by reduction of fracture
- Displaced and comminuted fractures in which the medial cortical buttress is not restored by reduction of the fracture

Type II: Reverse obliquity fractures

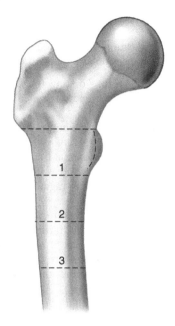

FIGURE 3.10 Fielding classification of subtrochanteric fractures [7]

Subtrochanteric Fractures

Fielding Classification (Fig. 3.10)

Based on the location of the primary fracture line in relation to the lesser trochanter.

Type I: At level of the lesser trochanter
Type II: <2.5 cm below the lesser trochanter
Type II: 2.5–5 cm below the lesser trochanter

Seinsheimer Classification (Fig. 3.11)

The Seinsheimer classification is based on the number of major bone fragments and the location and shape of the fracture lines.

Type I: Nondisplaced fracture or any fracture with <2 mm of displacement of the fracture fragments
Type II: Two-part fractures
           IIA: Two-part transverse femoral fracture
           IIB: Two-part spiral fracture with the lesser trochanter attached to the proximal fragment
           IIC: Two-part spiral fracture with the lesser trochanter attached to the distal fragment
Type III: Three-part fractures
           IIIA:Three-part spiral fracture in which the lesser trochanter is part of the third fragment, which has an inferior spike of cortex of varying length
           IIIB:Three-part spiral fracture of the proximal third of the femur, where the third part is a butterfly fragment
Type IV: Comminuted fracture with four or more fragments
Type V: Subtrochanteric-intertrochanteric fracture, including any subtrochanteric fracture with extension through the greater trochanter

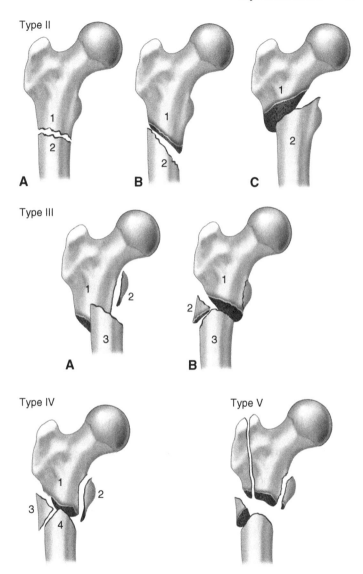

FIGURE 3.11 Seinsheimer classification [8]

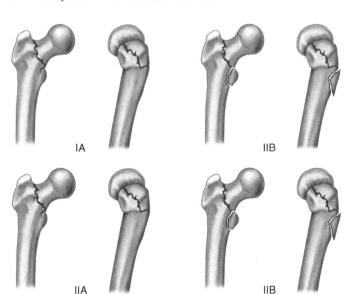

FIGURE 3.12 Russel-Taylor classification

Russel-Taylor Classification (Fig. 3.12)

Type I: Factures do not extend into piriformis fossa:
           IA: Lesser trochanter is attached to the proximal fragment
           IB: Lesser trochanter is detached from the proximal fragment

Type II: Fractures that extend into the piriformis fossa:
           IIA: No significant comminution or fracture of lesser trochanter.
           IIB: Significant comminution of the medial femoral cortex and loss of continuity of lesser trochanter

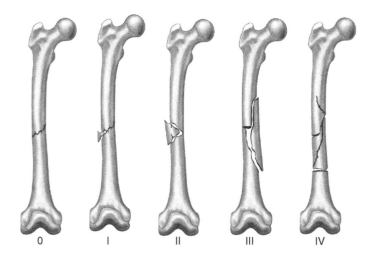

FIGURE 3.13 Winquist and Hansen classification of femoral shaft fractures: from left to right (*Type 0, Type I, Type II, Type III, Type IV*) [9]

Femoral Shaft

Descriptive Classification

- Open versus closed
- Location: proximal, middle, or distal one-third; supraisthmal or infraisthmal
- Pattern: spiral, oblique, or transverse
- Angulation: varus, valgus, or rotational deformity
- Displacement: shortening or translation
- Comminuted, segmental, or butterfly fragment

Winquist and Hansen Classification (Fig. 3.13)

Based on comminution; most useful for determining the need for interlocking nails.

Type I: Minimal or no comminution
Type II: Cortices of both fragments at least 50 % intact
Type III: 50–100 % cortical comminution
Type IV: Circumferential comminution with no cortical contact at the fracture site

Distal Femur

Descriptive Classification

- Open versus closed
- Location: supracondylar, intercondylar, condylar involvement
- Pattern: spiral, oblique, or transverse
- Articular involvement
- Angulation: varus, valgus, or rotational deformity
- Displacement: shortening or translation
- Comminuted, segmental, or butterfly fragment

AO Classification (Fig. 3.14)

A: Extraarticular
     A1: Simple, two-part supracondylar fracture
     A2: Metaphyseal wedge
     A3: Comminuted supracondylar fracture

B: Unicondylar
     B1: Lateral condyle, sagittal
     B2: Medial condyle, sagittal
     B3: Coronal

C: Bicondylar
     C1: Noncomminuted supracondylar "T" or "Y" fracture
     C2: Comminuted supracondylar fracture
     C3: Comminuted supracondylar and intercondylar fracture

Patellar Fractures

Descriptive Classification

- Open versus closed
- Displacement
- Pattern: stellate, comminuted, transverse, vertical (marginal), polar
- Osteochondral

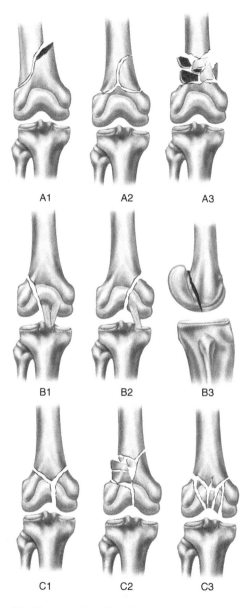

A1   A2   A3

B1   B2   B3

C1   C2   C3

FIGURE 3.14 Classification of the distal femur

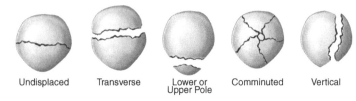

| Undisplaced | Transverse | Lower or Upper Pole | Comminuted | Vertical |

FIGURE 3.15 Saunders classification

Saunders Classification (Fig. 3.15)

Undisplaced
- Stellate
- Transverse
- Vertical

Displaced
  Noncomminuted
  ○ Transverse (central)
  ○ Polar (apical or basal)

  Comminuted
  ○ Stellate
  ○ Transverse
  ○ Polar
  ○ Highly comminuted

Knee Dislocations

Descriptive Classification (Fig. 3.16)

The position of the tibia relative to the femur defines the direction of dislocation.

Anterior: Forceful knee hyperextension beyond −30°; most common. Associated with posterior (and possibly anterior) cruciate ligament tear, with increasing incidence of popliteal artery disruption with increasing degree of hyperextension.

Posterior: Posteriorly directed force against proximal tibia of flexed knee; "dashboard" injury. Accompanied by anterior and posterior ligament disruption and popliteal artery compromise with increasing proximal tibia displacement.

Lateral: Valgus force. Medial supporting structures disrupted, often with tears of both cruciate ligaments.

Medial: Varus force. Lateral and posterolateral structures disrupted.

Rotational: Varus/valgus with rotatory component. Usually results in buttonholing of the femoral condyle through the articular capsule.

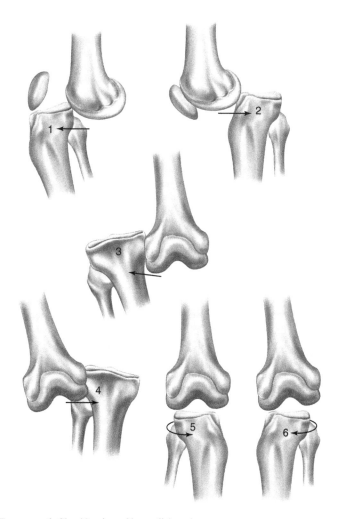

FIGURE 3.16 Classification of knee dislocations

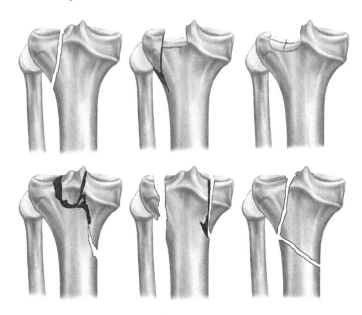

FIGURE 3.17 Schatzker classification of tibial plateau fractures [10]

Tibial Plateau Fractures

Schatzker Classification (Fig. 3.17)

Type I: Lateral plateaus, split fracture
Type II: Lateral plateau, split depression fracture
Type III: Lateral plateau, depression fracture
Type IV: Medial plateau fracture
Type V: Bicondylar plateau fracture
Type VI: Plateau fracture with metaphyseal-diaphyseal dissociation

Tibial/Fibular Shaft

Descriptive Classification

- Open versus closed
- Anatomic location: proximal, middle, or distal third
- Fragment number and position: comminution, butterfly fragments
- Configuration: transverse, spiral, oblique
- Angulation: varus/valgus, anterior/posterior
- Shortening
- Displacement: percentage of cortical contact
- Rotation
- Associated injuries

Gustilo and Anderson Classification of All Open Fractures

Type I
- Wound less than 1 cm long
- Moderately clean puncture, where spike of bone has pierced the skin
- Little soft tissue damage
- No crushing
- Fracture usually simple transverse or oblique with little omminution

Type II
- Laceration more than 1 cm long
- No extensive soft tissue damage, flap or contusion
- Slight to moderate crushing injury
- Moderate comminution
- Moderate contamination

Type III
- Extensive damage to soft tissues
- High degree of contamination
- Fracture caused by high velocity trauma

    IIIA: Adequate soft tissue cover
    IIIB: Inadequate soft tissue cover, a local or free flap is required
    IIIC: Any fracture with an arterial injury which requires repair

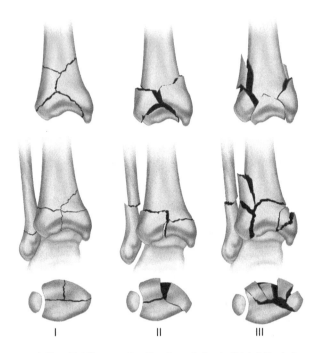

FIGURE 3.18 Ruedi-Allgower classification of distal tibial (pilon) fractures [11]

Pilon Fracture

Ruedi-Allgower Classification (Fig. 3.18)

Type 1:   No significant articular incongruity; cleavage fractures without displacement of bony fragments.
Type 2:   Significant articular incongruity with minimal impaction or comminution.
Type 3:   Significant articular comminution with metaphyseal impaction.

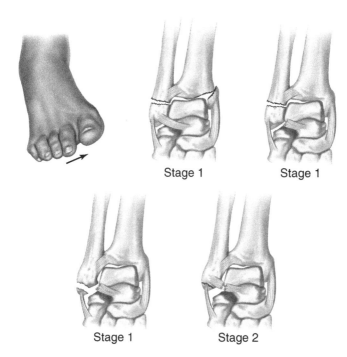

Stage 1   Stage 1

Stage 1   Stage 2

FIGURE 3.19 Lauge-Hansen classification of supination-adduction of the ankle

Ankle

Lauge-Hansen Classification (Fig. 3.19)

Four patterns, based on "pure" injury sequences, each subdivided into stages of increasing severity.

- Based on cadaveric studies
- Patterns may not always reflect clinical reality
- System takes into account the position of the foot at the time of injury and the direction of the deforming force

Supination-Aduction (SA)

Stage I: Transverse avulsion-type fracture of the fibula distal to the level of the joint or a rupture of the lateral collateral ligaments

Stage II: Vertical fracture of medial malleolus

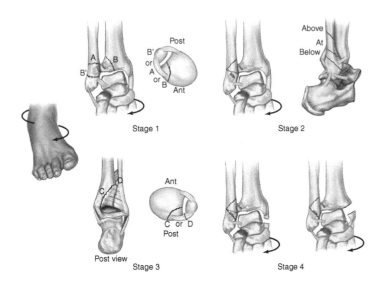

FIGURE 3.20 Lauge-Hansen classification of supination-external rotation of the ankle

Supination-External Rotation (SER) (Fig. 3.20)

Stage I: Disruption of the anterior tibiofibular ligament with or without an associated avulsion fracture at its tibial or fibular attachment.

Stage II: Spiral fracture of the distal fibula, which runs from anteroinferior to posterosuperior.

Stage III: Disruption of the posterior tibiofibular ligament or a fracture of the posterior malleolus.

Stage IV: Transverse avulsion-type fracture of the medial malleolus or a rupture of the deltoid ligament.

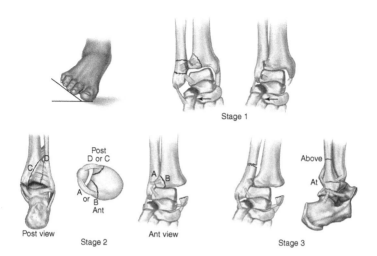

FIGURE 3.21 Lauge-Hansen classification of pronation-abduction of the ankle

Pronation-Abduction (PA) (Fig. 3.21)

Stage I: Transverse fracture of the medial malleolus or a rupture of the deltoid ligament.

Stage II: Rupture of the syndesmotic ligaments or an avulsion fracture at their insertions.

Stage III: Transverse or short oblique fracture of the distal fibula at or above the level of the syndesmosis.

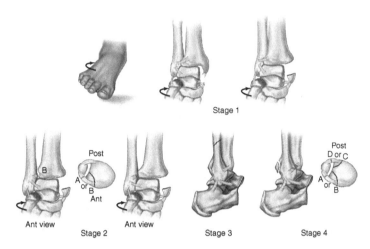

FIGURE 3.22 Lauge-Hansen classification of pronation-external rotation of the ankle

Pronation-External Rotation (PER) (Fig. 3.22)

Stage I: Transverse fracture of the medial malleolus or a rupture of the deltoid ligament.

Stage II: Disruption of the anterior tibiofibular ligament with or without an avulsion fracture at its insertion sites.

Stage III: Short oblique fracture of the distal fibula at or above the level of the syndesmosis

Stage IV: Rupture of the posterior tibiofibular ligament or an avulsion fracture of the posterolateral tibia.

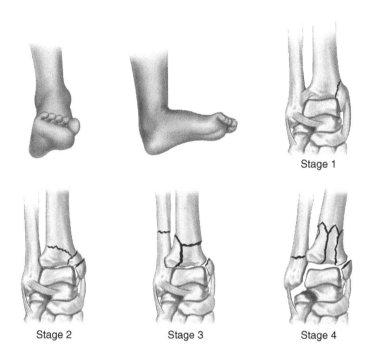

Stage 1

Stage 2   Stage 3   Stage 4

FIGURE 3.23 Lauge-Hansen classification of pronation-dorsiflextion of the ankle

Pronation-Dorsiflextion (PDA) (Fig. 3.23)

Stage I: Fracture of medial malleolus
Stage II: Fracture of anterior margin of tibia
Stage III: Supramalleolar fracture of fibula
Stage IV: Transverse fracture of posterior tibial surface

Danis-Weber Classification (Fig. 3.24)

Type A: Fibula fracture below the syndesmosis
          A1: Isolated
          A2: With fracture of medial malleolus
          A3: With posteromedial fracture
Type B: Fibula fracture at the level of syndesmosis
          B1: Isolated
          B2: With medial lesion (malleolus or ligament)
          B3: With medial lesion and fracture of posterolateral tibia
Type C: Fibula fracture above syndesmosis
          C1: Diaphyseal fracture of the fibula, simple
          C2: Diaphyseal fracture of the fibula, complex
          C3: Proximal fracture of fibula

Foot

Anatomic Classification of Talus Fractures

- Lateral process fractures
- Posterior process fractures
- Talar head fractures
- Talar body fractures
- Talar neck fractures

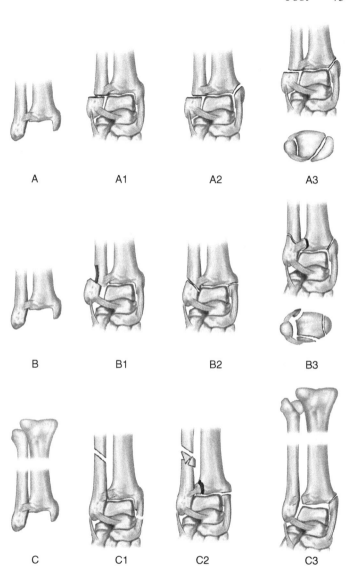

FIGURE 3.24 Danis-Weber classification [12]

Hawkins Classification of Talar Neck Fractures (Fig. 3.25)

Group I: Nondisplaced
Group II: Associated subtalar subluxation or dislocation
Group III: Associated subtalar and ankle dislocation
Group IV: Type III with associated talonavicular subluxation or
            dislocation (Canale and Kelley)

Calcaneal Fractures

Classification of Extraarticular Fractures

- Anterior process fractures: due to strong plantar flexion and inversion, which tightens the bifurcate and interosseous ligaments and leads to an avulsion fracture; alternatively, may occur with forefoot abduction with calcaneocuboid compression. Often confused with lateral ankle sprain; seen on lateral or lateral oblique views.
- Tuberosity fractures: due to avulsion by the Achilles tendon, especially in diabetics or osteoporotic women, or, rarely, may result from direct trauma; seen on lateral radiographs.
- Medial process fractures: vertical shear fracture due to loading of the heel in valgus; seen on axial radiograph.
- Sustentacular fractures: occur with heel loading accompanied by severe foot inversion. Often confused with medial ankle sprain; seen on axial radiograph.
- Body fractures not involving the subtalar articulation: due to axial loading. Significant comminution, widening, and loss of height may occur along with a reduction in the Bohler angle without posterior facet involvement.

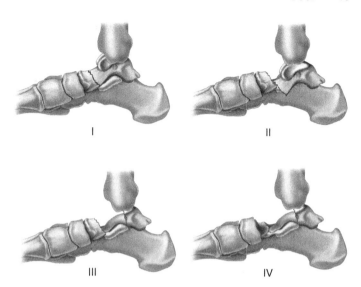

FIGURE 3.25 Hawkins classification of talar neck fractures

Essex-Lopresti Classification of Intraarticular Fractures (Fig. 3.26)

1. Fractures not involving subtalar joint

   (a) Tuberosity fractures:
   Beak type
   Avulsion of medial border
   Vertical
   Horizontal
   (b) Calcaneocuboid joint only:
   Parrot nose
   Various

2. Fractures involving subtalar joint

   (a) Without displacement
   (b) With displacement
   1. Tongue type
   2. Centrolateral depression type
   3. Sustantaculum tali fracture alone
   4. With gross comminution from below, sever tongue and joint depression type
   5. From behind forward with dislocation of subtalar joint

Souer and Remy Classification

Based on the number of bony fragments determined on Broden, lateral, and Harris axial views.
First degree: Nondisplaced intraarticular fractures
Second degree: Secondary fracture lines resulting in a minimum of three additional pieces, with the posterior main fragment breaking into lateral, middle, and medial fragments
Third degree: Highly comminuted

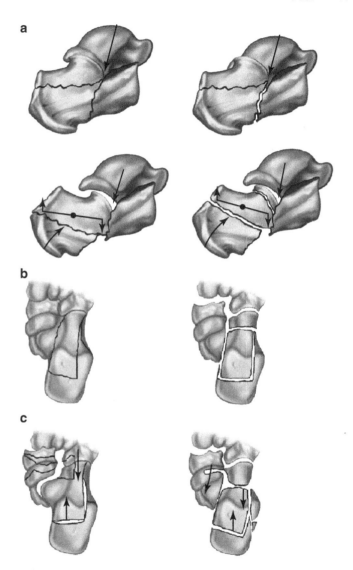

FIGURE 3.26 Essex-Lopresti classification of intraarticular fractures [13]

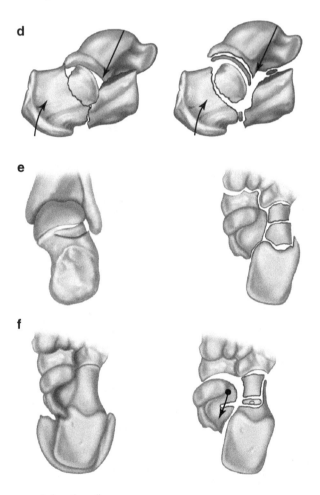

FIGURE 3.26 (continued)

Sanders Classification (Fig. 3.27)

- Classification based on the number and location of articular fragments as observed by computed tomography and found on the coronal image that shows the widest surface of the inferior facet of the talus.
- The posterior facet of the calcaneus is divided into three fracture lines (A, B, and C, corresponding to lateral, middle, and medial fracture lines, respectively, on the coronal image).

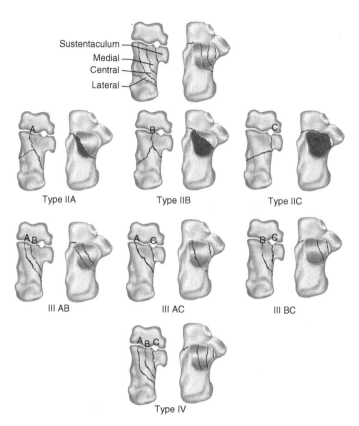

FIGURE 3.27 Sanders classification [14]

- Thus, a total of four potential pieces can result: lateral, central, medial, and sustentaculum tali.

Type I: All nondisplaced fractures regardless of the number of fracture lines

Type II: Two-part fractures of the posterior facet; subtypes IIA, IIB, IIC based on the location of the primary fracture line

Type III: Three-part fractures in which a centrally depressed fragment exists; subtypes IIIAB, IIIAC, IIIBC

Type IV: Four-part articular fractures; highly comminuted

Fractures of the Midfoot

Midtarsal Joint (Chopart Joint)

Main and Jowett Classification

1. Medial Stress Injury
   - This is an inversion injury with adduction of the midfoot on the hindfoot.
   - Flake fractures of the dorsal margin of the talus or navicular and of the lateral margin of the calcaneus or the cuboid may indicate a sprain.
   - In more severe injuries, the midfoot may be completely dislocated or an isolated talonavicular dislocation may occur. A medial swivel dislocation is one in which the talonavicular joint is dislocated, the subtalar joint is subluxed, and the calcaneocuboid joint is intact.
2. Longitudinal Stress Injury
   - Force is transmitted through the metatarsal heads proximally along the rays, with resultant compression of the midfoot between the metatarsals and the talus with the foot plantarflexed.
   - Longitudinal forces pass between the cuneiforms and fracture the navicular, typically in a vertical pattern.
3. Lateral Stress Injury
   - This s-called "nutcracker fracture" is a characteristic fracture of the cuboid as the forefoot is driven laterally, causing crushing of the cuboid between the calcaneus and the bases of the fourth and fifth metatarsals.
   - This is most commonly an avulsion fracture of the navicular with a comminuted compression fracture of the cuboid.
   - In more severe trauma, the talonavicular joint subluxes laterally and the lateral column of the foot collapses due to comminution of the calcaneocuboid joint.
4. Plantar Stress Injury
   - Plantarly directed forces may result in sprains to the midtarsal region with avulsion fractures of the dorsal lip of the navicular, talus, or anterior process of the calcaneus.
5. Crush Injuries

Navicular Fractures

Eichenholtz and Levin Classification

Type I: Avulsion fractures of tuberosity
Type II: A fracture involving the dorsal lip
Type III: A fracture through the body

Sangeorzan Classification (Fig. 3.28)

Type I: Transverse fracture line in the coronal plane, with no angulation of the forefoot
Type II: The major fracture line from dorsolateral to plantarmedial with talonavicular joint disruption and forefoot is displaced laterally.
Type III: Comminuted fracture pattern with naviculocuneiform joint disruption; associated fractures may exist (cuboid, anterior calcaneus, calcaneocuboid joints).

a

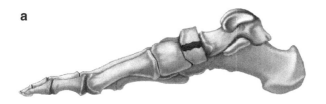

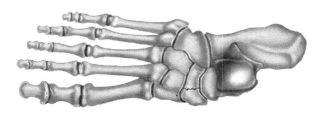

FIGURE 3.28 Sangeorzan classification. A, Type I; B, Type II; C, Type III. [15]

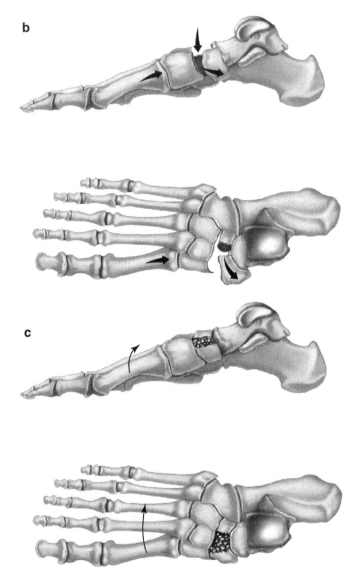

FIGURE 3.28 (continued)

Cuboid

OTA Classification of Cuboid Fractures

Higher letters and numbers denote more significant injury. Type A: extraarticular, no joint involvement

Type A: Extraarticular
              A1: Extraarticular, avulsion
              A2: Extraarticular, coronal
              A3: Extraarticular, multifragmentary
Type B: Partial articular, single joint (calcaneocuboid or cubotarsal)
              B1: Partial articular, sagittal
              B2: Partial articular, horizontal
Type C: Articular, calcaneocuboid and cubotarsal involvement
              C1: Articular, multifragmentary
                    C1.1: Nondisplaced
                    C1.2: Displaced

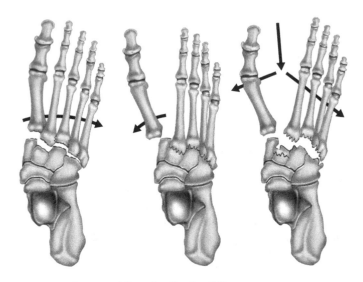

FIGURE 3.29 Quenu and Kuss classification [16]

Tarsometatarsal (Lisfranc) Joint

Quenu and Kuss Classification (Fig. 3.29)

Based on commonly observed patterns of injury.

Type 1: Homolateral. All five metatarsals displaced in the same direction

Type 2: Isolated: one or two metatarsals displaced form the others

Type 3: Divergent: displacement of the metatarsals in both the sagittal and coronal planes

Myerson Classification (Fig. 3.30)

A: Total incongruity
Lateral
Dorsoplantar

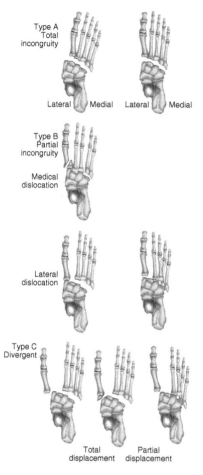

FIGURE 3.30 Myerson classification of Lisfranc fracture-dislocation [17]

B: Partial incongruity
     Medial
     Lateral

C: Divergent
     Partial
     Total

Fractures of the Base of the Fifth Metatarsal

Dameron & Lawrence & Boote classification
(Figs 3.31 and 3.32)

Zone 1:   Avulsion fractures
Zone 2:   Fractures at the metaphyseal-diaphyseal junction (Jone's fracture)
Zone 3:   Stress fractures of the proximal 1.5 cm of the shaft of the 5th metatarsal

First Metatarsophalangeal Joint

Bowers and Martin Classification

Grade I: Strain at the proximal attachment of the volar plate from the first metatarsal head
Grade II: Avulsion of the volar plate from the metatarsal head
Grade III: Impaction injury to the dorsal surface of the metatarsal head with or without an avulsion or chip fracture

Dislocation of the First Metatarsophalangeal Joint

Jahss Classification

Based on integrity of the sesamoid complex.

Type I: Volar plate is avulsed off the first metatarsal head; proximal phalanx displaced dorsally; intersesamoid ligament remains intact and lies over the dorsum of the metatarsal head.
Type IIA: Intersesamoid ligament is ruptured.
Type IIB: Longitudinal fracture of either sesamoid is seen.

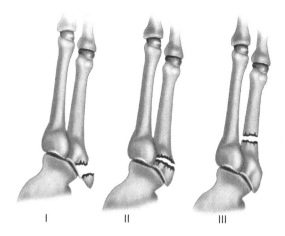

FIGURE 3.31 Dameron & Lawrence & Boote classification

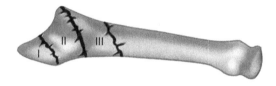

FIGURE 3.32 Dameron classification [18]

References

1. Young JWR, Burgess AR. Radiologic management of pelvic ring fractures. Baltimore: Urban & Schwarzenberg; 1987.
2. Letournel E, Judet R. Fractures of the acetabulum. New York: Springer; 1981.
3. Hansen S, Swiontkowski M. Orthopedic trauma protocols. New York: Raven; 1993. p. 238.
4. Garden RS. Low angle fracture of the femoral neck. J Bone Joint Surg. 1961;3-B:647–63.
5. Boyd HB, Griffin LL. Classification and treatment of trochanteric fractures. Arch Surg. 1949;58:853–66.
6. Ewans EM. The treatment of trochanteric fractures of the femur. J Bone Joint Surg Br. 1949;31-B:190–203.
7. Fielding JW, Magliato HJ. Subtrochanteric fractures. Surg Gynecol Obstet. 1966;122:555–60, now J Am Coll Surg.
8. Seinsheimer F. Subtrochanteric fractures of the femur. J Bone Joint Surg. 1977;60-A:300–6.
9. Winquist RA, Hansen ST. Comminuted fractures of the femoral shaft treated by interamedullary nailing. Orthop Clin North Am. 1980;11:633–48.
10. Schatzker J, McBroom R, Bruce D. The tibial plateau fracture: the Toronto experience 1968–1975. Clin Orthop. 1979;138:94–104.
11. Muller ME, Narzarian S, Koch P, et al. Manual of internal fixation. 2nd ed. New York: Springer; 1979. p. 279.
12. Muller ME, Nazarian S, Koch P. The AO classification of fractures. Berlin: Springer–Verlag; 1987.
13. Essex-Lopresti P. Mechanism, reduction techniques and results in fractures of the os calsis. Br J Surg. 1952;39:395–419.
14. Sanders R, Fortin P, Di Pasquale T, et al. Operative treatment in 120 displaced intraarticular calcaneal fractures. Clin Orthop. 1993;290:87–95.
15. Sangeorzan BJ, Benirschke SK, Mosca V, Mayo KA, Hansen Jr ST. Displaced intra-articular fractures of the tarsal navicular. J Bone Joint Surg Am. 1989;71A:1504–10.
16. Heckman JD, Bucholz RW, editors. Rockwood, green, and Wilkins' fractures in adults. Philadelphia: Lippincott, Williams & Wilkins; 2001.
17. Myerson MS, Fisher RT, Burgess AR, et al. Fracture-dislocations of the tarsometatarsal joints: end results correlated with pathology and treatment. Foot Ankle Int. 1986;6(5):228.
18. Dameron TB. Fractures of the proximal fifth metatarsal: selecting the best treatment option. J Am Acad Orthop Surg. 1986;3(2): 110–4.

Chapter 4
Fractures in Children

Salter-Harris Classification (Fig. 4.1)

Type I: Transphyseal fracture involving the hypertophic and calcified zones; prognosis is usually excellent, although complete or partial growth arrest may occur in displaced fractures.

Type II: Transphyseal fracture that exits the metaphysis; the metaphyseal fragment is known as the Thurston-Holland fragment; the periosteal hinge is intact on the side with the metaphyseal fragment; prognosis is excellent, although complete or partial growth arrest may occur in displaced fractures.

Type III: Transphyseal fracture that exits the epiphysis, causing intraarticular disruption; anatomic reduction and fixation without violating the physis are essential; prognosis is guarded because partial growth arrest and resultant angular deformity are common problems.

Type IV: Fracture that traverses the epiphysis and the physis, exiting the metaphysis; anatomic reduction and fixation without violating the physis are essential; prognosis is guarded, because partial growth arrest and resultant angular deformity are common.

Type V: Crush injury to the physis; diagnosis is generally made retrospectively; prognosis is poor because growth arrest and partial physeal closure commonly result.

Type VI: (Rang) Bruise or contusion to periphery of the epiphyseal plate. It can cause scaring, tethering, and arrest of the periphery of the epiphyseal plate, producing angular deformity.

S.B. Mostofi, *Fracture Classifications in Clinical Practice*
Second Edition, DOI 10.1007/978-1-4471-4420-5_4,
© Springer-Verlag London 2012

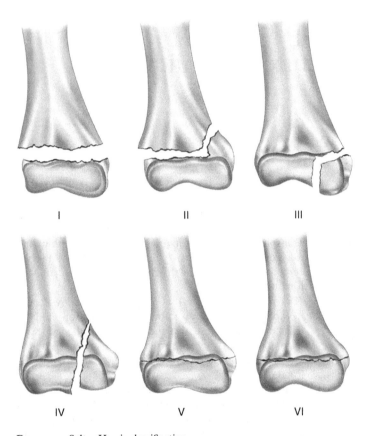

FIGURE 4.1 Salter-Harris classification

Supracondylar Humerus Fractures

Classification of Extension Type

Gartland Classification

Based on degree of displacement:
Type I: Nondisplaced
Type II: Displaced with intact posterior cortex; may be slightly angulated or rotated
Type III: Complete displacement; posteromedial or posterolateral

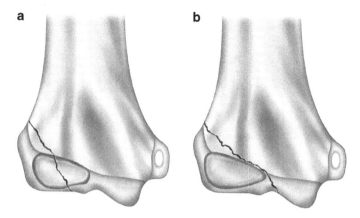

FIGURE 4.2 Milch classification [1]

Wilkins Modification of Gartland's Classification

Type 1:   Undisplaced
Type 2A: Intact posterior cortex and angulation only
   2B: Intact posterior cortex, angulation and rotation
Type 3A: Completely displaced, not cortical contact, posteromedial
   3B: Completely displaced, not cortical contact, posterolateral

Lateral Condylar Physeal Fractures

Milch Classification (Fig. 4.2)

Type I: Fracture line courses lateral to the trochlea and into the capitelotrochlear groove, representing a Salter-Harris type IV fracture. The elbow is stable because the trochlea is intact.
Type II: Fracture line extends into the apex of the trochlea, representing a Salter-Harris type II fracture. The elbow is unstable because the trochlea is disrupted.

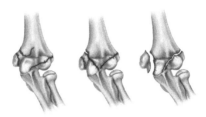

FIGURE 4.3 Kilfoyle classification [2]

Medial Condylar Physeal Fractures

Kilfoyle Classification (Fig. 4.3)

Type I: Impacted or greenstick fracture
Type II: A fracture through the humeral condyle into the joint
            with little or no displacement
Type III: An epiphyseal fracture that is intraarticular and involves the
            medial condyle with the fragment displaced and rotated

Transphyseal Fractures

Delee Classification

Based on ossification of the lateral condyle.

Group A: Infant, before appearance of lateral condylar ossification
          center (birth to 7 months of age); diagnosis easily missed;
          Salter-Harris type I.
Group B: Lateral condyle ossified (7 months to 3 years); Salter-
          Harris type I or II (fleck of metaphysis).
Group C: Large metaphyseal fragment, usually exiting laterally
          (ages 3–7 years).

T-Condylar Fractures

Wilkins and Beaty Classification

Type I: Nondisplaced or minimally displaced
Type II: Displaced, with no metaphyseal comminution
Type III: Displaced, with metaphyseal comminution

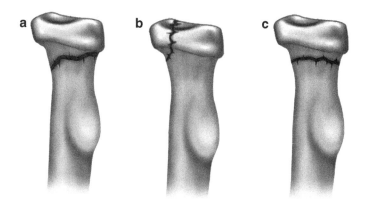

FIGURE 4.4 Wilkins classification of pediatric radial head and neck fractures

Radial Head and Neck Fractures

Wilkins Classification (Fig. 4.4)

Type A: Salter-Harris type I or II physeal injury
Type B: Salter-Harris type III or IV intraarticular injury
Type C: Fracture line completely within metaphysis
Type D: Fractures occurring when a dislocated elbow is being reduced
Type E: Fracture occurring with elbow dislocation.
    °   Fracture associated with elbow dislocation:
    Reduction injury
    Dislocation injury

Apophyseal Injuries of the Olecranon

Type I: Apophysitis
Type II: Incomplete stress fracture
Type III: Complete fractures
    A: Pure apophyseal avulsions
    B: Apophyseal-metaphyseal combinations

Pediatric Forearm

Descriptive Classification

Location: proximal, middle, or distal third

Type: plastic deformation, incomplete ("greenstick"), compression ("torus" or "buckle"), or complete
Displacement
Angulation
Associated physeal injuries: Salter-Harris types I to V

Distal Metaphyseal Fractures

Directional displacement

Dorsal
Volar

Fracture combination

Isolated radius
Radius with ulna
Ulnar styloid
Ulnar physis
Ulnar metaphysic, incomplete
Ulnar metaphysic, complete

Biomechanical patterns

Torus
Greenstick
One cortex
Two cortices
Complete fractures
Length maintained
Bayonet apposition

Letts Classification of Monteggia Fracture Dislocation (Fig. 4.5)

Dislocation of the radial head with fracture of ulna

1. Anterior bend
2. Anterior Greenstick
3. Anterior complete

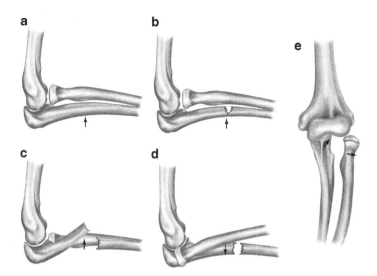

FIGURE 4.5 Letts classification of Monteggia fracture dislocation [3]

4. Posterior
5. Lateral

Walsh and McLaren Classification of Galeazzi Fracture Dislocation

Type I: Dorsal (apex volar) displacement of distal radius
           Radius fracture pattern
           Greenstick
           Complete
           Distal ulna physis
           Intact
           Disrupted (equivalent)

Type II: Volar (apex dorsal) displacement of distal radius
           Radius fracture pattern
           Greenstick
           Complete
           Distal ulna physis
           Intact
           Disrupted

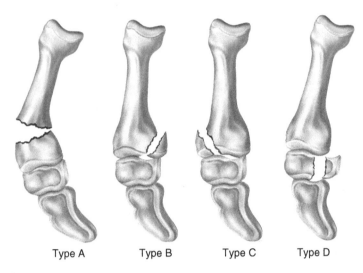

Type A   Type B   Type C   Type D

FIGURE 4.6 Classification of thumb metacarpal fractures

Scaphoid

Classification

Type A: Fractures of the distal pole
           A1: Extraarticular distal pole fractures
           A2: Intraarticular distal pole fractures

Type B: Fractures of the middle third
Type C: Fractures of the proximal pole

Classification of Thumb Metacarpal Fractures (Fig. 4.6)

Type A: Metaphyseal fracture
Type B: Salter-Harris type II physeal fractures with lateral
           angulation
Type C: Salter-Harris type II physeal fractures with medial
           angulation
Type D: Salter-Harris type III fracture (pediatric Bennett's
           fracture)

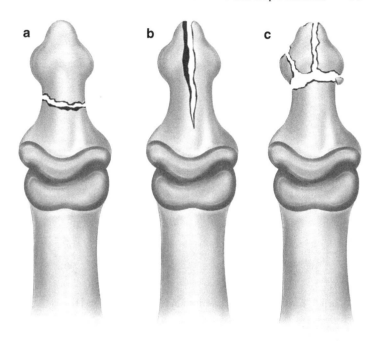

FIGURE 4.7 Extra epiphyseal fractures of the distal phalanx

Extra epiphyseal Fractures of the Distal Phalanx (Fig. 4.7)

A. Transverse diaphyseal fracture
B. Cloven-hoof longitudinal splitting fracture
C. Comminuted distal tuft fracture with radial fracture lines

Pediatric Pelvic and Hip Fractures (Fig. 4.8)

Torode and Zaeig Classification of Pelvic Fractures

1. Avulsion fractures
2. Iliac wing fractures

   (a) Separation of the iliac apophysis
   (b) Fracture of the bony iliac wing

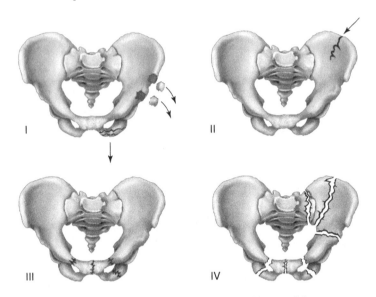

FIGURE 4.8 Torode and Zeig classification of pelvic fractures [4]

3. Simple ring fractures

    (a) Fractures of the pubis and disruption of the pubic symphysis
    (b) Fractures involving the acetabulum, without a concomitant ring fracture

4. Fractures producing an unstable segment (ring disruption fracture)

    (a) "Straddle fractures," characterized by bilateral inferior and superior pubic rami fractures
    (b) Fractures involving the anterior pubic rami or pubic symphysis and the posterior elements (e.g., sacroiliac joint, sacral ala)
    (c) Fractures that create an unstable segment between the anterior ring of the pelvis and the acetabulum

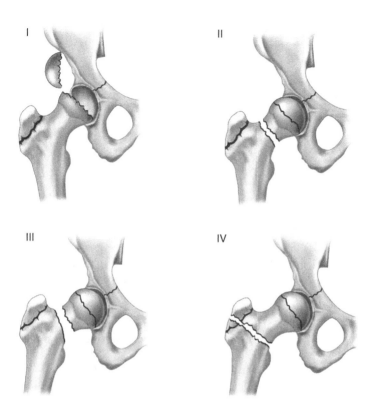

FIGURE 4.9 Classification of hip fractures in children [5]

Delbet Classification of Pediatric Hip Fractures (Fig. 4.9)

Type I: Transepiphyseal fracture
Type II: Transcervical fracture
Type III: Cervicotrochanteric fracture
Type IV: Intertrochanteric fracture

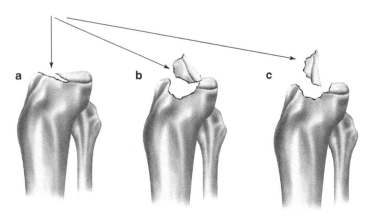

FIGURE 4.10 Meyers and McKeever classification

Tibial Spine (Intercondylar Eminence) Fractures

Meyers and McKeever Classification (Fig. 4.10)

Type I: Minimal or no displacement of fragment
Type II: Angular elevation of anterior portion with intact poste-
            rior hinge
Type III: Complete displacement with or without rotation

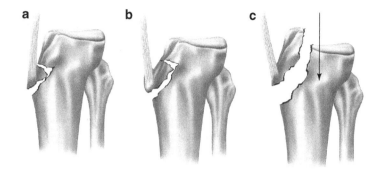

FIGURE 4.11 Watson-Jones classification of tibial tuberosity fractures

Tibial Tuberosity Fracture

Watson-Jones Classification (Fig. 4.11)

Type I: A small fragment, displaced superiorly
Type II: A larger fragment involving the secondary centre of ossification and proximal tibial epiphysis
Type III: A fracture that passes proximally and posteriorly across the epiphyseal plate and proximal articular surface of tibia (Salter-Harris Type III)

Calcanial Fractures

Schmidt and Weiner Classification of Calcanial Fractures

Type I:

(a) Fracture of the tuberosity of aphophyses
(b) Fracture of the sustentaculum
(c) Fracture of the anterior process
(d) Fracture of the anterior inferolateral process
(e) Avulsion fracture of the body

Type II: Fracture of the posterior and/or superior parts of the tuberosity

Type III: Fracture of the body not involving the subtalar joint
Type IV: Nondisplaced or minimally displaced fracture through the subtalar joint
Type V: Displaced fracture through the subtalar joint

   (a) Tongue type
   (b) Joint depression type

Type VI: Either unclassified or serious soft-tissue injury, bone loss, and loss of the insertions of the Achilles tendon.

References

1. Milch H. Fractures and fracture dislocations of the humeral condyles. J Trauma. 1964;4:592–604.
2. Kilfoyle RM. Fractures of the medial condyle and epicondyle of the elbow in children. Clin Orthop Relat Res. 1965;41:43–50.
3. Walsh HPJ, McLaren CAN, Owen R. Galeazzi fractures in children. J Bone Joint Surg Br. 1987;69B:730–3.
4. Torode I, Zieg D. Pelvic fractures in children. J Pediatr Orthop. 1985;5(1):76–84.
5. Rockwood Jr CA, Wilkins KE, Beaty JH, editors. Rockwood and Green's fractures in children, vol. 3. 4th ed. Philadelphia: Lippincott-Raven; 1996. p. 1151.

Chapter 5
Periprosthetic Fractures

Periprosthetic Shoulder Fractures

University of Texas at San Antonio Classification (Fig. 5.1)

Type I: Fractures occurring proximal to the tip of the humeral prosthesis

Type II: Fractures occurring in the proximal portion of the humerus with distal extension beyond the tip of the humeral prosthesis

Type III: Fractures occurring entirely distal to the tip of the humeral prosthesis

Type IV: Fractures occurring adjacent to the glenoid prosthesis

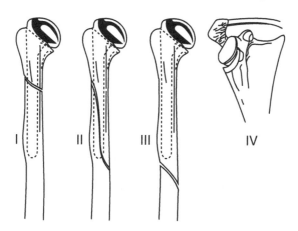

FIGURE 5.1 Periprosthetic fracture of the shoulder [1]

S.B. Mostofi, *Fracture Classifications in Clinical Practice*
Second Edition, DOI 10.1007/978-1-4471-4420-5_5,
© Springer-Verlag London 2012

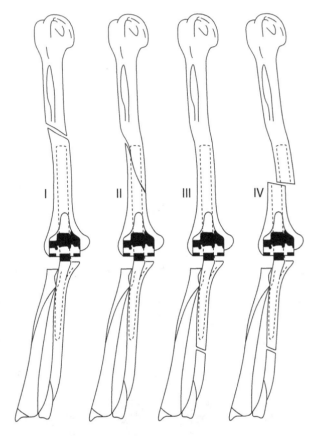

FIGURE 5.2 Periprosthetic elbow fractures [2]

Periprosthetic Elbow Fractures (Fig. 5.2)

Classification

Type I: Fracture of the humerus proximal to the humeral component.

Type II: Fracture of the humerus or ulna in any location along the length of the prosthesis.

Type III: Fracture of the ulna distal to the ulnar component.

Type IV: Fracture of the implant.

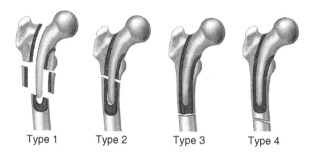

FIGURE 5.3 Cooke and Newman classification of periprosthetic fracture about total hip implants [3]

Periprosthetic Hip Fractures

Vancouver Classification (Duncan and Masri)

Type A: Involve the trochanteric area
   AG: Involve the greater trochanter
   AL: Involve the lesser trochanter
Type B: Fractures around the stem or extending slightly distal to it
   B1:   Implant well fixed
   B2:   Implant loose, bone stock adequate
   B3:   Implant loose, bone stock inadequate
Type C: Fractures distal to the stem that the presence of the femoral component may be ignored.

Johansson Classification

Type I: Fracture proximal to prosthetic tip with the stem remaining in the medullary canal
Type II: Fracture extending beyond distal stem with dislodgement of the stem from the distal canal
Type III: Fracture entirely distal to the tip of the prosthesis

Cooke and Newman (Modification of Bethea) (Fig. 5.3)

Type I: Explosion type with comminution around the stem; the prosthesis is always loose, and the fracture is inherently unstable
Type II: Oblique fracture around the stem; fracture pattern is stable, but prosthetic loosening usually is present

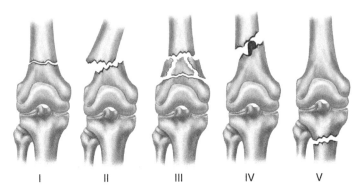

FIGURE 5.4 Periprosthetic fracture of the knee [4, 5]

Type III: Transverse fracture at the distal tip of the stem; the fracture
            is unstable, but prosthetic fixation is usually unaffected
Type IV: Fracture entirely distal to prosthesis; fracture is unstable,
            but prosthetic fixation is usually unaffected

Periprosthetic Knee Fractures

Femoral Fractures

Lewis and Rorabeck Classification

Type I: Undisplaced fractures, prosthesis intact
Type II: Displaced fractures, prosthesis intact
Type III: Displaced or undisplaced fracture, prosthesis loose or
            failing

Neer Classification, with Modification by Merkel (Fig. 5.4)

Type I: Minimally displaced supracondylar fracture
Type II: Displaced supracondylar fracture
Type III: Comminuted supracondylar fracture
Type IV: Fracture at the tip of the prosthetic femoral stem of the
            diaphysis above the prosthesis
Type V: Any fracture of the tibia

Tibial Fractures (Neer and Merkel Type V)

Goldberg Classification

Type I: Fractures not involving cement/implant composite or
             quadriceps mechanism
Type II: Fractures involving cement/implant composite and/or
             quadriceps mechanism
Type IIIA: Inferior pole fractures with patellar ligament
             disruption
Type IIIB: Inferior pole fractures without patellar ligament
             disruption
Type IV: Fracture-dislocation

Ortiguera and Berry Classification for Periprosthetic Patella Fractures

Type I: Intact extensor mechanism and a stable implant
Type II: Disruption of the extensor mechanism with or without a
             stable implant
Type III: Intact extensor mechanism and a loose implant
    IIIA: Reasonable remaining bone stock
    IIIB: Poor bone stock

References

1. Rockwood CA, Green DP, Bucholz RW, Heckman JD. Rockwood
   and Green's fractures in adults. 4th ed. Philadelphia: Lippincott-
   Raven; 1996. p. 543.
2. Heckman JD, Bucholz RW, editors. Rockwood, Green, and Wilkins'
   fractures in adults. Philadelphia: Lippincott Williams & Wilkins;
   2001.
3. Cooke PH, Newman JH. Fractures of the femur in relation to
   cemented hip prostheses. J Bone Joint Surg Br. 1988;70B:386.
4. Neer C, Grantham S, Shelton M. Supracondylar fracture of the adult
   femur. A study of 110 cases. J Bone Joint Surg Am. 1967;49A:591.
5. Merkel KD, Johnson Jr EW. Supracondylar fracture of the femur
   after total knee arthroplasty. J Bone Joint Surg Am. 1986;68A:
   29–43.

Index

S.B. Mostofi, *Fracture Classifications in Clinical Practice*   109
Second Edition, DOI 10.1007/978-1-4471-4420-5,
© Springer-Verlag London 2012